Woodmill High School Library

KT-433-589

This book is to be returned on or before
the last date stamped below.

18710

1 3 SEP 1996	2 0 DEC 2002
- 4 OCT 1996	22 APR 2003
1 6 OCT 1998	27 OCT 2003
2 9 JAN	- 8 JUL

DRUGS

AND

SPORT

CHRISTIAN WOLMAR

Wayland

DRUGS AND CRIME
DRUGS AND THE MEDIA
DRUGS AND MEDICINE
DRUGS AND SPORT

Designer Helen White
Series editor Deborah Elliott

Cover Steroid abuse is considered to be rife among body builders.
The drugs enable athletes to train harder and longer thus building up muscles. Unfortunately, however, the side effects – acne, liver disease and even cancer – negate the benefits.

First published in 1992 by
Wayland (Publishers) Ltd.
61 Western Road, Hove, East Sussex BN3 1JD

British Library Cataloguing in Publication Data
Wolmar, Christian
Drugs and Sport. – (Drugs)
I. Title II. Series
362.293088796
ISBN 0 7502 0317 X

Typeset by White Design
Printed by Canale C.S.p.A in Turin

CONTENTS

18710
613.83

Woodmill High School Library
Dunfermline

CHAPTER ONE

WINNING IS EVERYTHING

CANADIAN sprinter Ben Johnson was disqualified for drug-taking from the Seoul Olympics in 1988 after 'winning' the 100 m. His fall from grace brought the use of drugs in sport into public prominence once and for all. Modern sport is now so highly competitive and, except in the few sports that remain amateur, potentially so profitable, that many athletes find it difficult to resist the temptation to improve themselves in any way possible, both illegal and legal.

The use of drugs appears to be concentrated in specific sports. In some, such as weightlifting and cycling, drug-taking has been very widespread at times. In others, like tennis, cricket and soccer, so far there have been virtually no drugs scandals.

Since the earliest days of sport, athletes have looked at ways to improve their performances; drugs have been an obvious choice for that extra competitive edge. The ancient Greeks, the forerunners

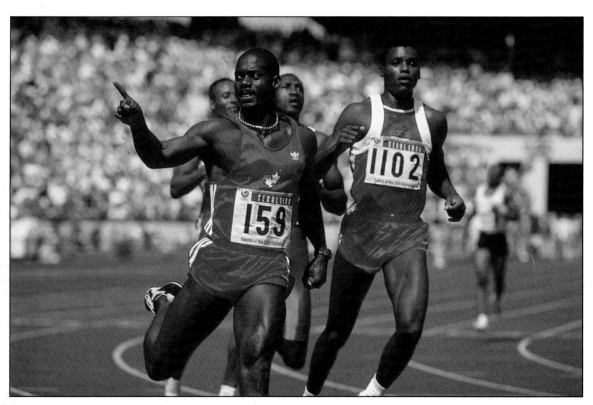

Number one in the world! But not for long. Amid the glare of the world's media, Ben Johnson was stripped of his 100 m Olympic title in 1988 after failing a drugs test.

of today's Olympic athletes, tried a variety of ways of enhancing their performances. For example, wrestlers often ate as much as 4.5 kg of lamb a day to build up their bodies. Some athletes apparently ate special mushrooms which were thought to help them mentally. Others drank a concoction of horses' hooves boiled in oil to give their performances a boost.

As sport became popular in the nineteenth century, there were many reports of drug use. In one of the first recorded instances, canal swimmers who raced in Amsterdam in 1865 were alleged to have used various substances to help them keep going. Around the same time, some cyclists who went in for very long endurance tests, were known to use mixtures of heroin and cocaine.

The most famous early case is that of Tommy Hicks, the winner of the 1904 marathon at the Olympic Games in St Louis, USA. He made no secret of the fact that he had been given several doses of strychnine (which is very poisonous but acts as a stimulant in small quantities) and brandy to keep him on his feet during the race. There were no rules about drug use and not only did Hicks keep his medal, but he said, despite collapsing at the finish, *'I would rather have won this race than be president of the USA.'*

While there was undoubtedly some drug use by sportsmen and women

Throughout history athletes have experimented with different ways to improve their performances. Some ancient Greek wrestlers are believed to have eaten up to 4.5 kg of lamb a day to build up their strength.

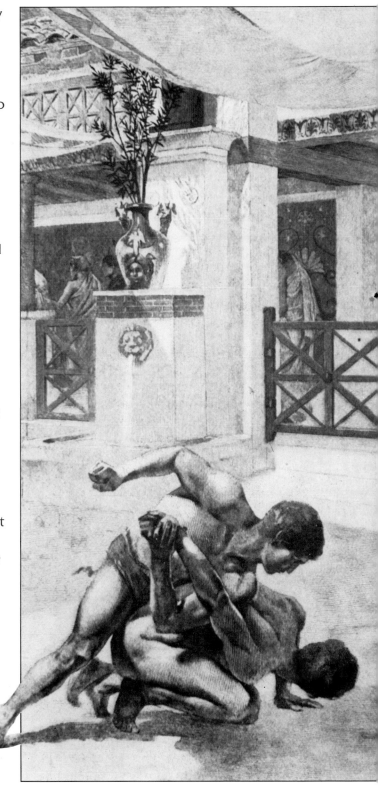

throughout the twentieth century, the issue did not come to prominence again until the mid 1950s, when France attempted to control drugs in sport. Other countries followed suit, spurred on by the death of Danish cyclist, Knut Jensen, at the 1960 Rome Olympics. He had taken a stimulant and collapsed in the fierce Italian heat. Another cyclist, Britain's Tommy Simpson, became the first to die of drug-related problems in the full glare of the world's television during the 1967 Tour de France. He was climbing a mountain on a very hot day and died as a result of stress caused by the amphetamines he had taken (see chapter 5). A previous winner of the Tour de France, Jacques Anquetil, said at the time that it was 'practically impossible' for top cyclists not to use stimulants (such as amphetamines).

The incident forced the world's sporting bodies to take notice. The International Olympic Committee (IOC) set up a medical committee in 1967 which banned certain drugs. It defined 'doping' as '*the use of substances or techniques in any form or quantity alien or unnatural to the body with the exclusive aim of obtaining*

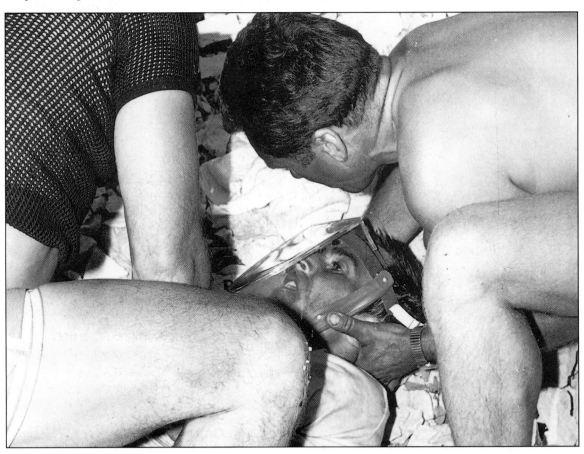

British cycling champion Tommy Simpson collapsed mysteriously during the 1967 Tour de France. He died later in Avignon Hospital as a result of stress caused by amphetamines.

Anabolic steroids – the most widely used types of drug among sportsmen and women – has been banned since the mid 1970s.

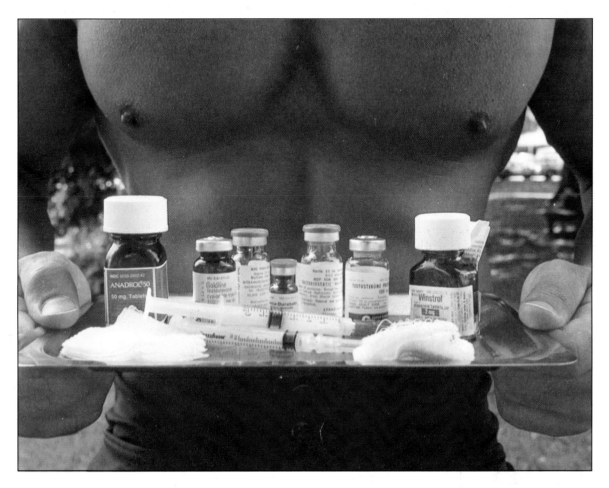

an artificial or unfair increase of performance in competition.' As we shall see later (chapter 3), it is a controversial definition because there are all kinds of techniques and training practices which could be considered as equally unethical as the use of drugs. One early problem about imposing bans was the difficulty of testing for drugs as there were very few laboratories able to carry them out. Anabolic steroids, one of the most widely used types of drug in sport, was not even banned until the mid 1970s when a test was finally developed for it.

At the 1968 Mexico Olympics testing was only carried out for 'research' purposes and the results did not effect the athletes concerned. Indeed the only meaningful tests were those carried out to determine whether all the female competitors were biologically women. At the 1967 European Games, Polish sprinter Eva Klubokowska had failed the screening. Also, at the 1968 Olympics, much comment was made over the fact that the famous Soviet shot putting sisters, Tamara and Irina Press, did not turn up, presumably for fear of failing the tests.

The talented Soviet shot put champion Tamara Press and her sister Irina did not attend the 1968 Mexico Olympics, despite being strong medal hopes. Their absence fuelled speculation that the two 'women' were concerned about the sex test which would prove if they were biologically female.

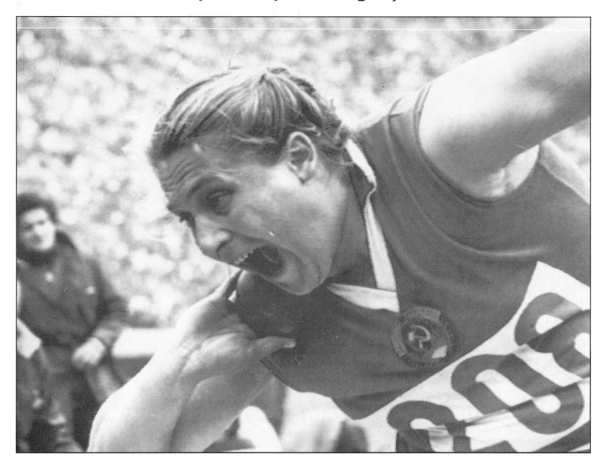

Throughout the 1970s and 1980s, controls on doping increased. More drugs were added to the banned list, and lifetime bans began to be imposed in some sports (see chapter 3). However, drug use by some athletes grew. In Britain, an inquiry by the British Amateur Athletic Board in 1988 estimated that one in ten British athletes might have used banned substances at some time. Many people believe the figure for world-wide use is much higher. In 1985, Daley Thompson, the British decathlete, said that as many as 30 per cent of British and 80 per cent of US international athletes had used drugs to improve their performances. Yet, testing revealed a much smaller percentage. In 1987, of 37,882 samples taken throughout the world only 854 were found to be positive (just 2.25 per cent). Many of these positive results were for drugs which had been taken for genuine medical purposes, such as cough mixtures and asthma sprays. Another problem, of course, is that athletes use drugs during training and stop several weeks before they are due to compete. It is a dangerous game of cat and mouse.

There are some signs that the controls are beginning to take effect. The British Sports Council reported a drop in the number of positive samples between 1989 and 1990, despite an increase in the number of samples taken. Whether that is the result of athletes being more clever about their use of drugs or whether it reflects a real decrease is impossible to know or even to find out.

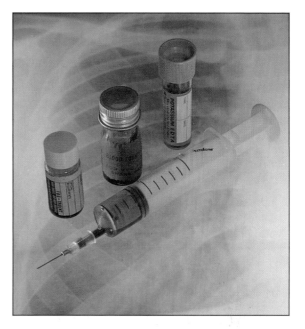

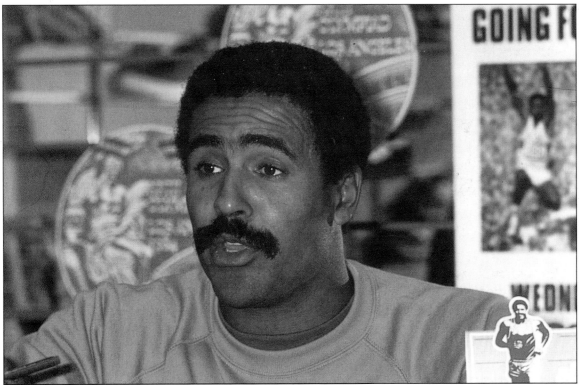

ABOVE **Decathlete Daley Thompson is very outspoken about the use of drugs in sport. In 1985 he claimed that about 80 per cent of US international athletes had used drugs.** TOP RIGHT **Syringe and sample bottles used for taking and testing blood samples.**

CHAPTER TWO

TYPES AND EFFECTS

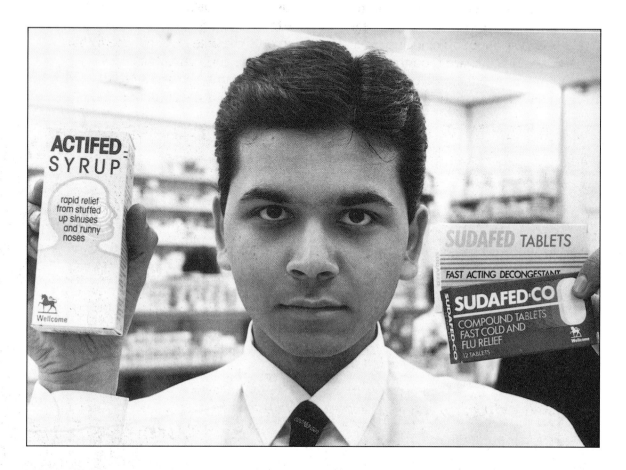

THERE are now so many banned drugs that it is difficult to know what is included. Many athletes genuinely make mistakes by taking drugs for medical ailments. Some drugs are banned completely, while others are allowed for medical treatment. Some naturally occurring chemicals, such as testosterone, are allowed in the body up to certain levels but result in a ban if detected in larger quantities.

There are now six categories of drugs on the IOC's banned list and four classes of drugs 'subject to certain restrictions'.

A pharmacist shows some of the products containing banned Olympic drugs that can be bought over the counter in most countries.

The IOC also bans 'blood doping' and substances which change the composition of urine in attempts to disguise the presence of drugs (both explained in the next chapter).

Anabolic steroids are generally thought to be the most widely used drug. They are synthetic (manufactured rather than natural) male hormones, originally invented to help human tissue grow back after burning accidents. Anabolic means 'building up'. Athletes use steroids, in combination with extra training and more food, to build up their muscles. At least half a dozen sportspeople, including a British body builder, are thought to have died from the effects of steroids. These effects include acne, liver disease, internal bleeding, sexual problems and possibly even cancer. Typically, steroids increase aggression, allowing athletes to train harder and longer, thereby building their muscles and pushing them to better performances. Steroids can change a person's character, making them more aggressive and combative.

One commonly used steroid, testosterone, is a natural hormone.

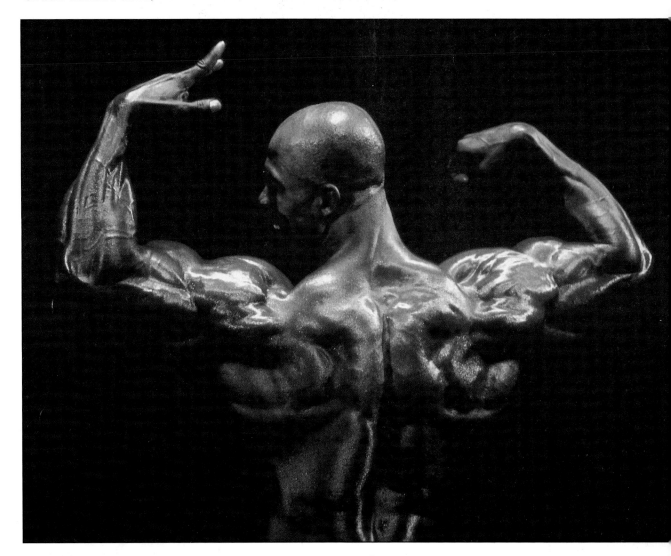

Steroid abuse is thought to be particularly rife among body builders because the drugs enable them to train harder and build up muscles.

Athletes must not have over six times the average natural level. The problem for the administrators is that if they set the legal limit too high, then people can get away with taking low doses. However, if they set it too low, people who naturally have a large amount in their bodies will, quite unfairly, fall foul of the regulations.

The most widely used steroid is called methandrostenalone (sold as dianabol), for which the annual unlicensed sales in the USA are thought to be more than US $100 million. Ben Johnson used a steroid called stanozolol (stromba).

Anabolic steroids help athletes in sports that require muscular strength.

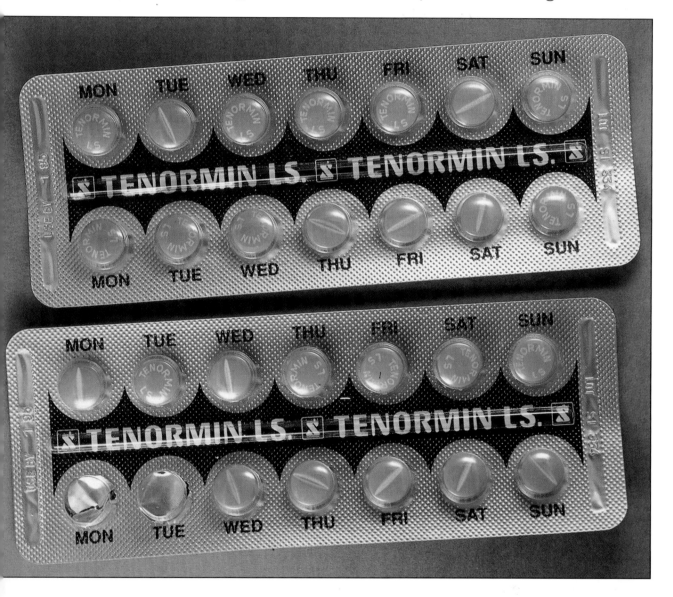

Blister packs of Tenormin LS, a type of beta blocker. This drug is used to treat angina (a heart condition) and to lower blood pressure. Athletes use beta blockers to relax.

Weightlifting, American football and field sports such as shot putting and hammer throwing are obvious examples, but as Ben Johnson showed, they can also help sprinters.

Stimulants are the second most common drug found in testing. They can reduce fatigue and increase alertness and competitiveness. Several sportspeople have died as a result of stimulant use, most notably Tommy Simpson (see Chapter 5). The body can build up tolerance quite easily to amphetamines, which means that increased doses have to be used to achieve the same effect.

Because many common remedies for colds and flu contain stimulants, athletes must never use such products without first checking with a doctor. Otherwise they could find that they have used a banned substance by mistake.

Stimulants are potentially attractive to athletes in many different sports. Cyclists use them to keep going on long rides, while runners feel stimulants help them run faster as they can tolerate pain much better. However, they are of no use when precision skills are needed, such as in soccer or hockey, because they tend to produce loss of judgement.

Beta blockers have been banned only recently. They were developed to treat heart conditions by reducing the effect of stress on the body and lowering the heart beat, effectively allowing it to rest more which is helpful for people with bad hearts. Until recently their use was permitted if prescribed by a doctor. For example, at the 1984 Olympics in Los Angeles, every member of the modern pentathlon teams had a beta blocker prescription. By 1988 beta blockers had been banned and a Spanish athlete was disqualified from the pentathlon at the Seoul Olympics in 1988 for using them.

Because beta blockers slow down the heart rate and reduce tension, they are particularly useful for athletes in sports which require intense concentration such as archery, shooting and snooker. Even ski jumpers used them to relax. Snooker authorities resisted banning beta blockers but were persuaded to do so for the image of the sport.

Narcotic analgesics, or more simply painkillers, are drugs which reduce pain. Most induce sleep, too, and therefore are not very useful to athletes. However, according to the IOC, there is evidence *'that narcotic analgesics have been and are abused in sports'*. The Committee points out that there are major side effects, most notably the high risk of addiction.

The main benefit of narcotic analgesics is that they allow athletes to train or compete in spite of painful injuries. They can also be used to reduce the risk of cramp. One unusual use has been cyclists who find the 'rush effect' of the drug (the initial surge of energy immediately after it has been taken) helps them through the last few moments of a sprint finish.

Regulations on nartcotic analgesics are very complicated. Some of these drugs, such as corticosteroid painkillers, are allowed. They can be taken by inhalation or applied on the skin and can even be injected into the artery as long as the IOC has been notified in advance by the athlete's team doctor.

There are two other groups of drugs on the IOC's banned list, diuretics (covered in the next chapter) and peptide hormones and analogues - a variety of drugs which, for example, include a growth hormone originally developed to prevent dwarfism

There are many different types of drugs available and others are being developed all the time. Sports administrators are finding it increasingly difficult to work out which to ban.

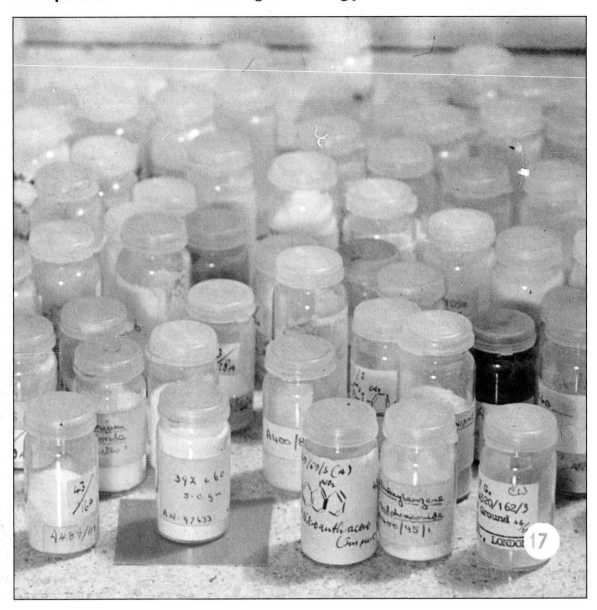

in children but which may help body building. Given to boys before puberty, it could also increase their growth, making them well over 1.8 m tall and with enormous hands, feet, ears and noses.

Within each group of drugs, there are many types of preparation developed for various uses, and which contain different doses of each chemical. New preparations are being developed by drugs manufacturers all the time. All this adds to the complexity of the task facing sports administrators when deciding which substances to ban and which to allow.

CHAPTER THREE

THE DILEMMAS FACING SPORT

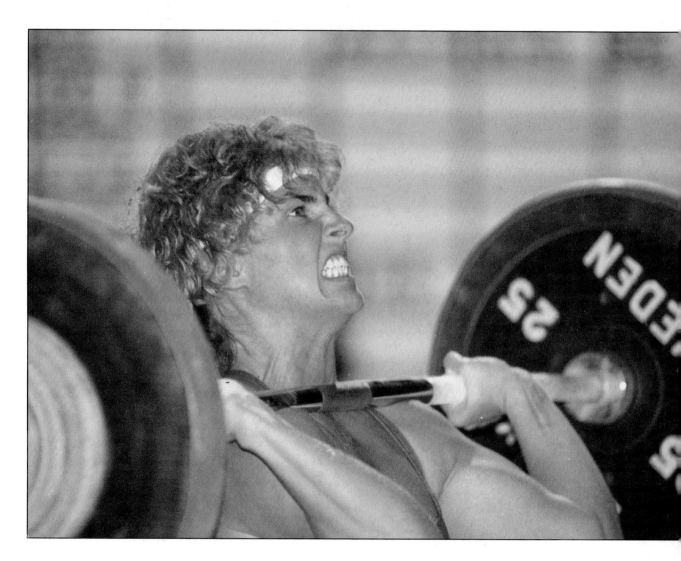

THE sporting authorities were slow to respond to the increased use of drugs in sports. There was growing evidence in the late 1950s and early 1960s that the problem was widespread. However, it was not until the 1970s that testing began to be carried out and only in the 1980s did it

Body building, powerlifting and weightlifting are considered to have the largest number of drug abusers. Most athletes do not resort to 'chemical assistance' but those that do tarnish the image of their sports.

become widely accepted. In the early 1960s, for example, the British Amateur Weightlifting Association, pressed the Sports Council (association to promote sport) to take action against the dangers of anabolic steroids. Even now, there are still differences between the punishments meted out by different countries and particularly among different sports.

Many sporting bodies were reluctant to act. Any publicity about the use of drugs in sport goes against the clean image of sporting activity. The health-promoting picture of fit, young sportsmen and

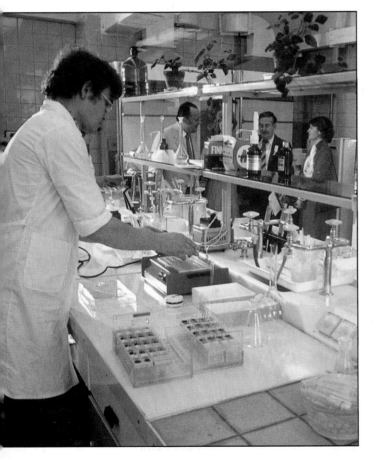

Testing for anabolic steroid use at the Moscow Olympics in 1980. Tests were first introduced in Montreal in 1976.

women competing against each other is made less attractive by the idea that nasty little pills or even nastier injections are responsible for the athletes' performances. The mere association of drugs with sport was likely to reduce the potential for sponsorship, stop people from attending sports events and generally tarnish the clean sports image. If they turned a blind eye to the problem, then maybe it would just go away. It didn't.

There was also the problem of coming up with efficient and reliable tests at a reasonable price, particularly for the most widely used group of drugs, anabolic steroids. Previously, there had been no medical need for a test but, with the encouragement of sporting bodies, two new ways of testing for steroids were worked out by 1973.

There was also a long debate by doctors about whether or not drugs did improve athletes' performances. Doctors were worried that if they admitted publicly that anabolic steroids, in particular, lead to much better athletic performances, then it would encourage even more athletes to take these drugs.

The tests were carried out first at the 1976 Olympic Games in Montreal, Canada. Although relatively few proved positive - only eight out of 275 - this did not mean that athletics had necessarily become 'clean'. Athletes had learned to use drugs during their training programmes but not too close to competitions. This meant that all traces had disappeared from their bodies by the time they competed. Also, many had used testosterone, which, because it was found in the body naturally, was not tested for at that time. By 1982, the IOC had added testosterone to its banned list.

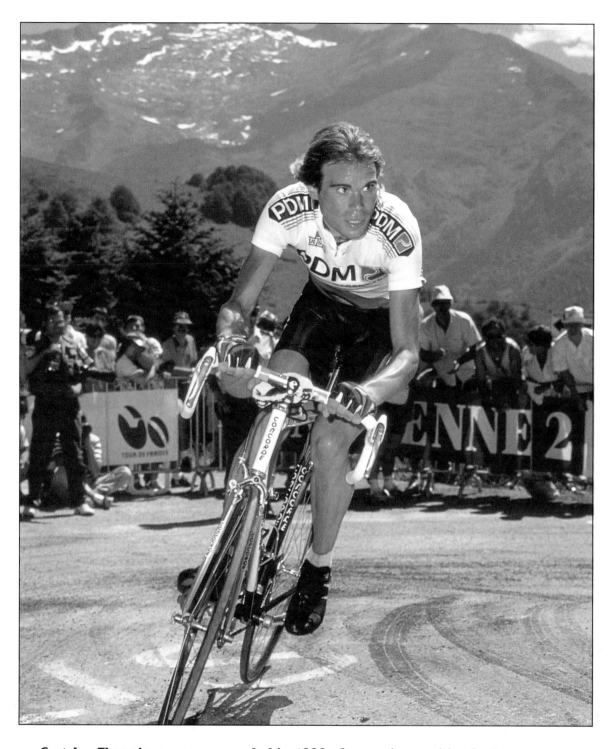

Gert-Jan Theunisse was suspended in 1990 after testing positive for testosterone three times. The Dutch cyclist protested his innocence claiming he had a naturally high level of the male hormone.

There are still no tests for some drugs, such as human growth hormone, EPO (see chapter 8). While they can be detected, they are always present in the body and because the amount they occur varies between individuals, the sporting bodies have found it impossible to set a level at which their presence becomes illegal.

There have been several disputes over these drugs. The Dutch cyclist Gert-Jan Theunisse, for example, was suspended in 1990 for twelve months after having tested positive for testosterone three times within two years. He protested his innocence, arguing that he had a naturally higher level of testosterone in his body than normal.

Analysing blood samples in a laboratory.

BLOOD DOPING

There is another technique used by athletes for which testing is very difficult to detect - blood doping. Some athletes have blood removed some weeks or months before a competition, which means their own supply will be replenished naturally by the body. Then, just before the competition, the old blood is injected back, thereby increasing the athletes' blood supplies. The idea is that with more blood, the body will be able to carry more oxygen. However, doctors are not certain if there is any benefit to be obtained. Another alternative is simply to have a blood transfusion of someone else's blood shortly before the competition. At least one litre is needed to improve performance.

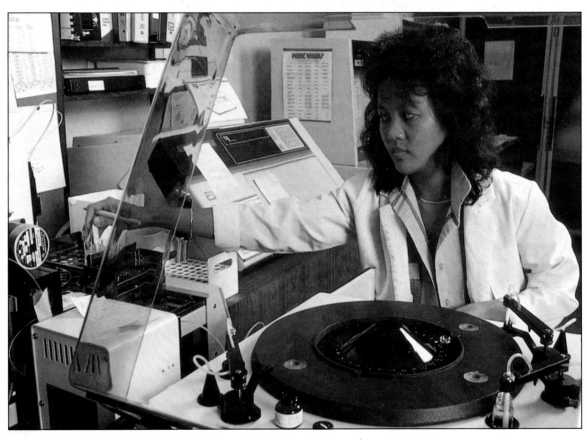

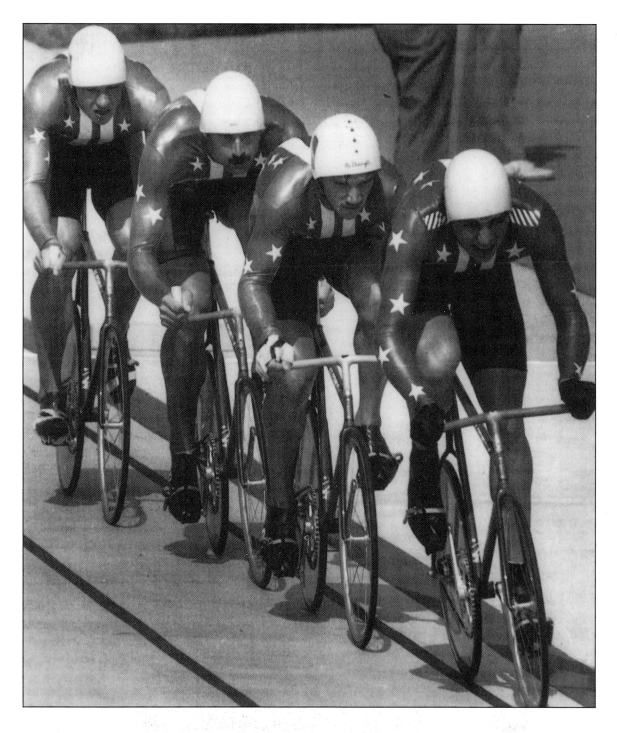

Four members of the US cycling team during competition at the Los Angeles Olympics in 1984. In an interview with the *New York Times* a physician named three of the four cyclists pictured as having been involved in a blood transfusion process known as blood doping.

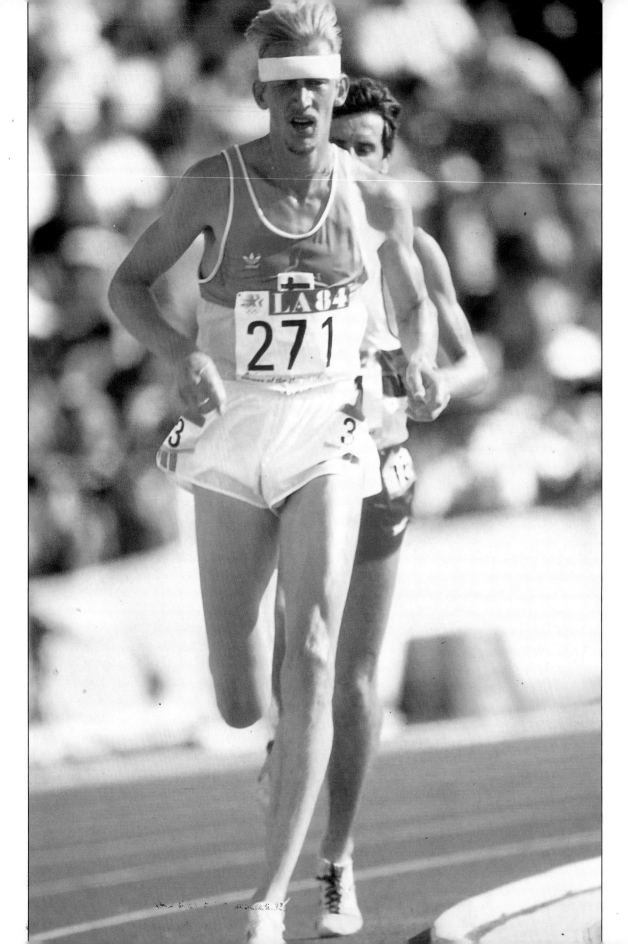

At the 1984 Los Angeles Olympics, the winning US cycling team made no secret of the fact that they had used blood doping, which at the time was legal. Ironically, at the same Games, the Finnish 10,000 m runner, Martti Vainio, was discovered to have taken steroids only because he also used blood doping. The blood had been taken and stored while he was on steroids but, despite the fact that he had stopped taking drugs before the Games, the old blood showed up positive in the tests and he was stripped of his silver medal.

Blood doping has since been banned. Tests for blood doping have been devised and were carried out first at the 1989 Nordic Skiing World Championships. The test developed for use in skiing competitions involves checking the age of blood in the body. Blood is replenished automatically by the body within three months. Therefore if a high proportion of old blood is found in the system, it is clear that blood doping has been used. Similarly, the test can ascertain whether the competitor has had a recent blood transfusion.

Some athletes, like the US sprinter and long jumper Carl Lewis, would like blood testing for all events. The problem is that the test is carried out by taking a blood sample and many athletes are worried about the risk of contracting AIDS from dirty needles. Some athletes may also have religious objections to having blood removed from their bodies.

There is also concern about the cost. One blood test costs US $250 and many sporting bodies, particularly those from developing countries, could not afford to carry out blood tests. All drug testing is currently carried out on urine which is

18710
613.83

OPPOSITE Martti Vainio, the Finnish 10,000 m runner, had his silver medal from the Los Angeles Olympics taken away when it was discovered he had used blood doping.

BELOW Carl Lewis has called for blood testing to be carried out in all events.

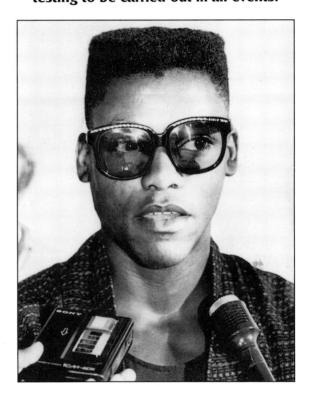

much easier for administrators to deal with than blood testing, which requires more equipment and trained medical staff.

The problems and difficulties over testing are shown by the fact that some drugs are banned for reasons other than because they help an athlete's performance. For example, diuretics, which make people urinate and therefore eject substances from their bodies more quickly are banned, as are 'masking agents' which are used to try to cover up the presence of other drugs.

Woodmill High School Library
Dunfermline

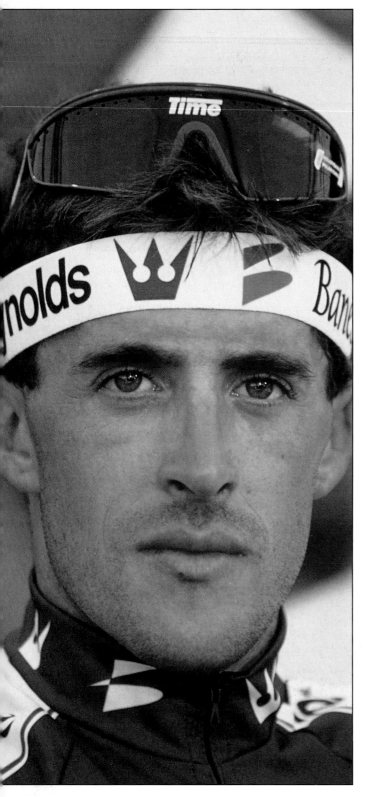

The drug-taking athletes are often one step ahead of the authorities. Pedro Delgado, the cyclist who won the 1988 Tour de France, was found to have traces of probecinide, a masking agent for anabolic steroids. Although, at the time, the drug was banned by the IOC, the cycling authorities only banned it after the race. Delgado kept his title.

Another dilemma is over the use of drugs genuinely taken for medical purposes. Beta blockers, for example, are widely used by people with heart complaints. As one snooker player put it, *'If I stop taking it* (inderal, a beta blocker), *I would be giving myself a long term death sentence'*. Similarly, asthma sufferers are often prescribed drugs which contain banned doping substances, such as adrenalin and ephedrine. However, in most cases alternatives are available or an athlete can get permission prior to a competition to take a particular drug.

There is another irony over the use of illegal drugs, such as cannabis. While most of the drugs banned by the sporting authorities are legal and have medical uses, most sporting authorities have no rules about marijuana, a substance that is illegal virtually everywhere.

Spanish cyclist Pedro Delgado narrowly escaped disqualification from the 1988 Tour de France because although traces of probecinide were found in his body, the drug was not banned by cycling authorities. Probecinide is a masking agent for anabolic steroids. The drug was banned by the IOC, however. The cycling authorities decided to ban probecinide after this incident.

CHAPTER FOUR

TESTS AND PUNISHMENTS

ALONG with the problem of coming up with tests for all banned drugs, authorities have to decide when to carry them out. In most sports, the first three in any competition and a few other random competitors are tested. That is no longer good enough. Tests have to be carried out between competitions as well as during them, particularly when checking for anabolic steroid use. The problem is that competitors stop taking the drugs a few weeks before the event and hope that all traces of the drugs have left their bodies' systems. They will still benefit from the drugs' abilities to help them build up their muscles.

The British Amateur Weightlifting Association, conscious that the sport has been increasingly associated with drug taking, especially since Bulgarian, Spanish

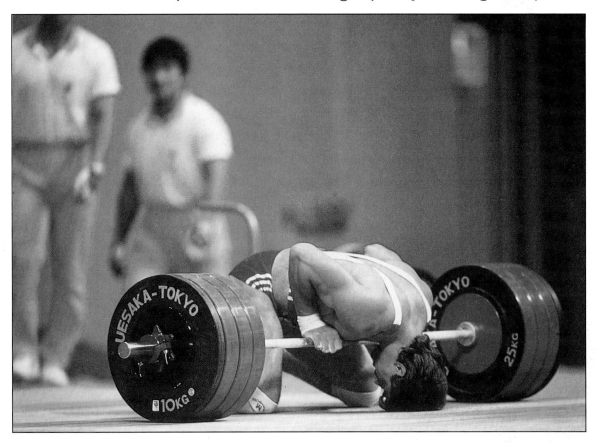

Weightlifting associations around the world have taken strict measures to try to clean up the image of the sport.

and Hungarian weightlifters were sent home from the 1988 Seoul Olympics, has devised very strict rules. Its members must be available at all times for random testing, even to the extent that they have to give telephone numbers when they are not at home for any length of time. Anybody refusing to take a test, or deliberately not being available for one without a good excuse, is automatically banned for life. The Association is also looking at the possibility of using tests which show up positive even four or five months after the athlete has stopped using drugs, rather than the few weeks which the current tests are good for. According to Wally Holland of the British Amateur Weightlifting Association, there are concerns that forcing people to be in constant contact with the Association is an infringement of personal liberties. But, he says, 'nobody forces them to join the Association and become a weightlifter. They can take up tiddlywinks instead.'

Random testing during training, rather than before competitions, has also been introduced in athletics and other sports are likely to follow suit.

HOW TESTS WORK

Competitors who are selected to be tested are required to provide urine samples divided into two, A and B. These samples are passed through a machine called a gas chromatograph/mass spectrometer. As the complicated name implies, this is really two machines in one. The first separates the various substances that make up the sample, and the second identifies what they are. After the chemicals are separated, they are bombarded with high-energy ions which break them up, creating unique chemical fingerprints. These are then checked

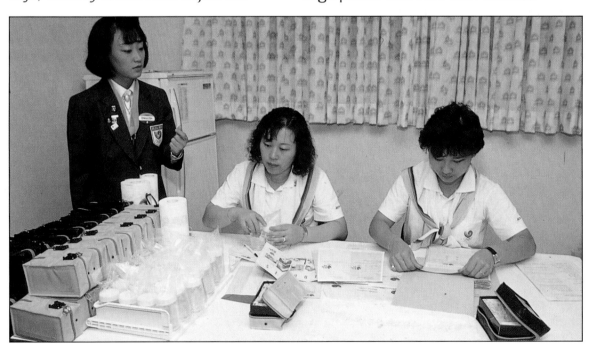

Processing urine samples prior to testing at the Seoul Olympics in 1988.

against a database of known compounds. The system used at the 1988 Seoul Olympics could compare 70,000 different compounds in less than one minute and the manufacturer claimed that it could detect concentrations as low as one part per million. As an article in the *Daily Telegraph* put it, *'that is equivalent to detecting traces from a teaspoonful of sugar after it has been deposited and circulated in an Olympic swimming pool'*.

When a banned substance is found a portion of the sample is tested again to eliminate the possibility of error. Then, if the result is positive, the second - 'B' - jar is brought out and tested in the presence of the athlete, his or her coach and doctor. If still positive, the athlete goes to a hearing of the sporting body to provide an explanation.

PUNISHMENT

There is a fierce debate among both competitors and the sporting authorities about how severe punishments should be. Banning people for life from competing in their sport is obviously the highest penalty. However, it can easily lead to problems - unlucky athletes who take the wrong cough mixture before a race, for example, may find themselves never able to compete again.

Currently, there is an established punishment 'tariff' in athletics, which is the minimum that must be applied by any country competing in international competition. For using anabolic steroids, amphetamines, cocaine and peptide hormones and analogues, the penalty for the first use is a two-year ban, and for any subsequent use a life ban. For using stimulants, such as caffeine and narcotic analgesics, such as codeine, the penalties

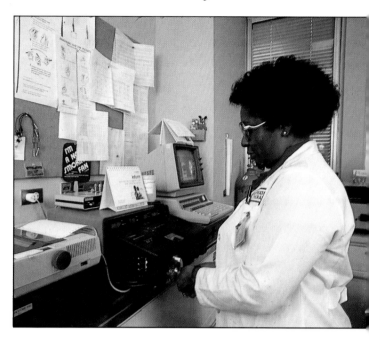

A technician feeds blood samples into a machine to be analysed.

are less - a ban of three months for the first offence, two years for the second and life for the third.

When Martti Vainio, the Finnish runner, was discovered to have taken anabolic steroids, his ban ended up being just eighteen months and there were complaints from many sports administrators that this was not severe enough. The hardliners argue that without an effective deterrent - and a ban from the sport is the only possible one since the drugs are mostly legal - sportsmen and women will continue to risk the chance of detection for the opportunity to become top of their sports. Those arguing for lesser penalties say that harsh penalties simply take out of the sport many fine athletes who may have succumbed to temptation or simply been unlucky to have been one of the many using drugs to have been caught. (See final chapter for discussion.)

CHAPTER FIVE

CAUGHT OUT

MANY famous competitors, from across the world, have been found to have used drugs. Others have paid the ultimate penalty, dying in circumstances which point to drugs as the cause.

TOMMY SIMPSON

Britain has had very few famous cyclists. Tommy Simpson was one of the best, becoming an international star in the 1960s after winning stages in the world's greatest cycle race, the Tour de France. Many people considered him a possible future winner.

Simpson had been doing well, lying seventh in the 1967 Tour de France, when he came to Mont Ventoux. This involved a climb of almost 2,000 m. The temperature was unbearable, possibly as high as 50°C according to some commentators. Simpson was struggling, looking bemused, as he climbed up to near the summit. His body finally gave out, and he fell off his bike. He was helped back on to it by spectators. He quickly collapsed again, and went into a coma. Simpson died a few hours later in hospital. His last words had been spoken at the roadside,

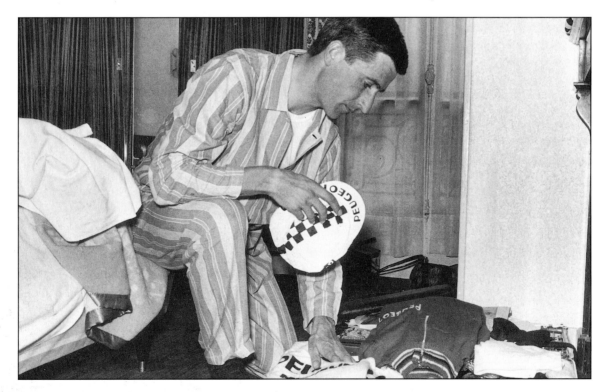

Cyclist Tommy Simpson who died in 1967 amid allegations of drug abuse.

26

'Put me back on my bike. Go on, go on'. His death shocked the world as it was in the full glare of the television cameras that capture every moment of the race.

Simpson's death provoked a fierce debate over whether drugs had been involved. The race director, Jacques Goddet, said that it was not *'entirely natural'* that an experienced competitor should die while racing.

There has never been any conclusive proof that Simpson died from drug use. Two empty tubes were found in his jersey pocket and a third contained two different kinds of drugs. Furthermore, traces of amphetamine and another drug were found in his body but it is not sure whether the drugs actually killed him or whether he had a weak heart anyway. The post mortem examination found that he had died of heart failure, caused by heat exhaustion, lack of oxygen (because of the height) and overwork.

DIEGO MARADONA

There have been few recorded incidents of drug use in soccer. Association soccer players don't need the big muscles that anabolic steroids build up, and the skills required on the ball would make the use of amphetamines counter-productive. But Diego Maradona, the world's most famous, and in the 1980s undoubtedly the world's best, soccer player succumbed to the temptations of drugs taken for so-called 'pleasure' and 'fun' - cocaine was his undoing.

The stocky little midfield player had grown up in the slums of Buenos Aires, capital of Argentina. His genius was quickly noticed and he became a professional footballer at the age of fifteen. He came to Europe to play first for

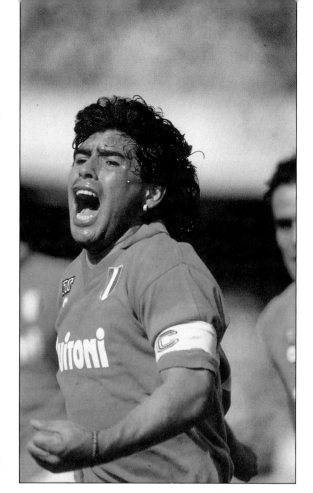

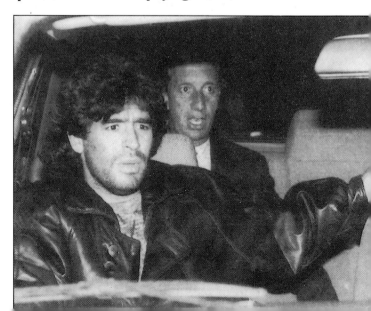

ABOVE **Diego Maradona on top of the world during his days with Napoli. His career took a dramatic turn for the worst when he was charged with the possession and distribution of drugs. He is pictured** BELOW **leaving a Buenos Aires police station after paying a $20,000 bail.**

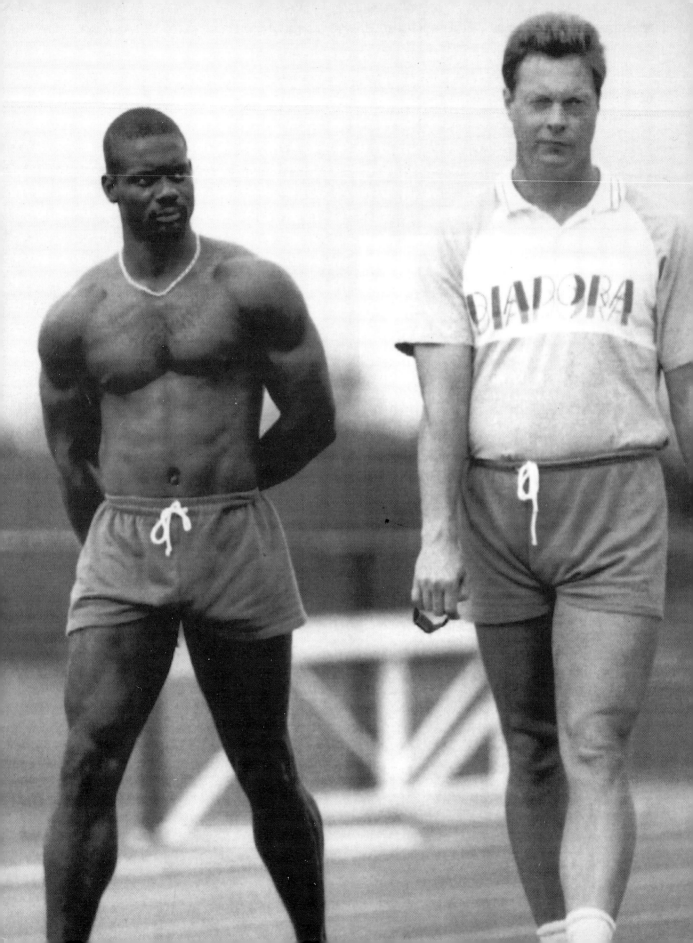

Barcelona in Spain and then, for a fee of £5 million, for Napoli in Italy. He was being paid £1.2 million per year, and earnt three times that much in sponsorship and other commercial deals. Maradona brought success to the club - Napoli won its first championship for decades. The Argentinian became a local hero and was idolized by soccer fans around the world. His playboy life-style, however, led to him being caught up in several infamous sex and drugs scandals.

In March 1991, he was tested for drugs after a match against Bari and was found to have traces of cocaine. There were allegations of involvement in cocaine dealing rings and at one time there was even an arrest warrant out for him. Maradona returned home to Argentina. He was suspended for two years by the Italian Federation, a decision then endorsed by the international federation, FIFA. It meant that Maradona could not play anywhere in the world. The glittering career of the thirty year-old genius seemed to be over.

BEN JOHNSON

Undoubtedly, the most famous sports drugs scandal involved Ben Johnson. When the Canadian sprinter won the 100 m at the Seoul Olympics, the world was elated by his explosive running. The 100 m is the most prestigious race of all and there was widespread admiration for the Jamaican-born Johnson. He already held the 100 m world record but he broke that again in winning the race. As one newspaper ironically put it, *'only a urine sample stood between Ben Johnson and a place in history'*.

However, the urine sample proved positive, finding traces of a steroid called

OPPOSITE Ben Johnson (left) and his coach Charlie Francis are shown in this 1988 photograph during training at Toronto's York University. Francis had recently told the Dublin Inquiry, investigating the Johnson affair, that the Canadian sprinter had begun taking steroids in 1981.

BELOW Johnson testifying at the Dublin Inquiry.

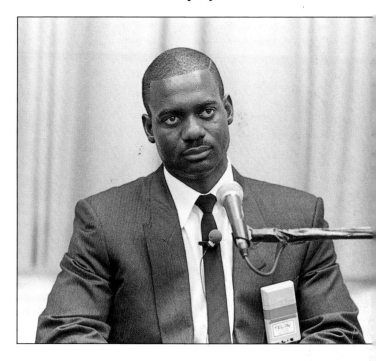

stanozolol. Johnson was stripped of his gold medal and his world record. At first he denied having used drugs, giving a number of bizarre excuses: a drink he had taken before the race was 'spiked', the tests had been faked. Later his doctor was to confess to having given Johnson drugs over a number of years. Johnson was even said to have used them before setting the world record in Rome in 1987.

Johnson received a two-year ban. When he started running again he could never match the form that had made him the champion. At the inquiry by the Canadian Government into the Johnson affair, several people involved gave evidence to suggest that drugs were widely used by Canada's athletes. Ben Johnson's coach, Charlie Francis, said that 80 per cent of top flight athletes used drugs. Angella Issajenko, the country's top female sprinter, set out a staggering list outlining her ten-year programme of 'chemical training'. Johnson's doctor said that the athlete had used a drug that could not be detected by laboratories within a week or ten days of its use. He claimed to have been very surprised when Johnson tested positive because he had previously been tested when using drugs and no traces had shown up. The question raised by all this evidence is whether Johnson was merely unlucky to be caught or whether he was genuinely one of the few athletes to use drugs.

BIRGIT DRESSEL

The kind of dreadful cocktail of drugs taken by some athletes in seeking to become champions is illustrated by the tragedy of Birgit Dressel, a heptathlete from what was then West Germany. Heptathletes have a particularly demanding programme. They have to compete in seven different disciplines, ranging from the shot put and the javelin to the 100 m hurdles and 800 m. Therefore it demands an unequalled range of strength and speed which Dressel decided to obtain through using no less than twenty different drugs. She is believed to have had 400 injections of body-building drugs and there is little doubt that they helped her improve her performance. Between 1984 and 1986 she rose from twenty-sixth in the world to sixth, but in 1987 she died after suffering a massive allergic reaction to the combination of drugs she had taken.

No single drug could be blamed for her death but the combination, for some unknown reason, proved to be lethal.

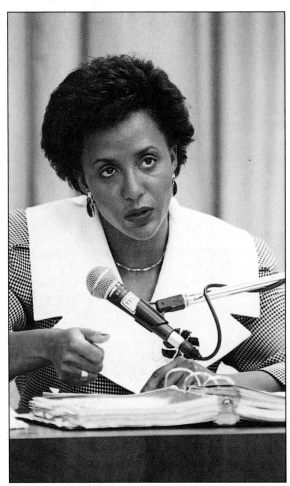

ABOVE Angella Issajenko, Johnson's team-mate, testified at the Dublin Inquiry. The sprinter admitted to having used drugs for ten years.

OPPOSITE West German heptathlete Birgit Dressel died in agony aged twenty-six after an unbelievable programme of drug abuse.

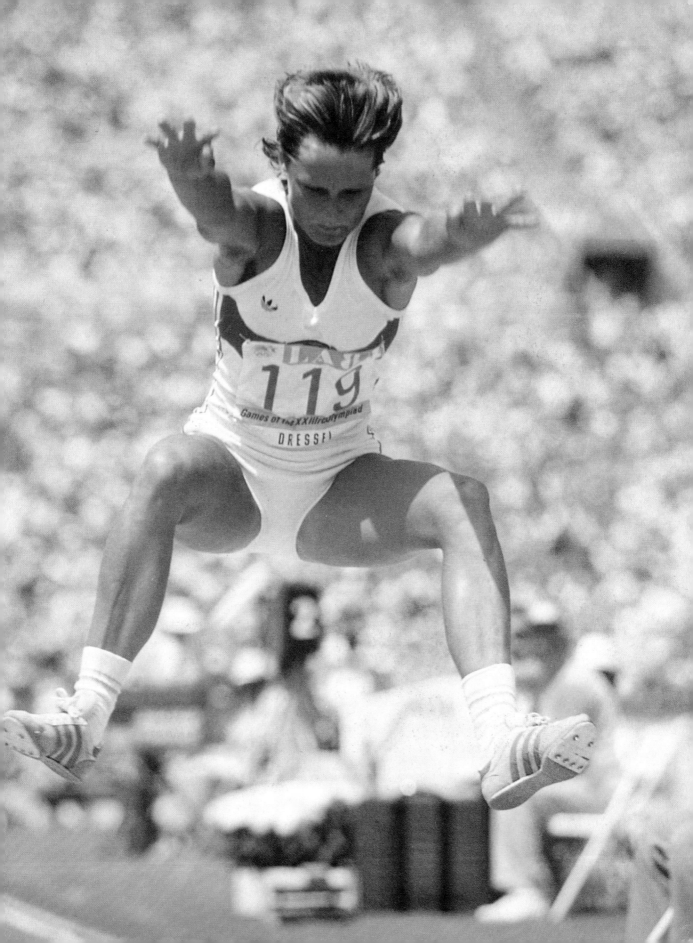

CHAPTER SIX

DRUGS FOR SALE

THERE appears to be two main sources of drugs – doctors and coaches who work with athletes, and dealers who often operate out of gymnasiums. It is, of course, a shady, often illegal, world and therefore there are no reliable statistics. However, one estimate suggests that US $100 million worth of one particular steroid is used by US sportsmen and women every year. There is a lot of money to be made out of them.

Athletes who have used drugs in the past and now regret it are often ready to talk openly about their experiences. Other evidence about this underground world can also be obtained from those caught smuggling or selling the drugs. Steroids, the most commonly used drug, can be obtained legally in both Britain and the US only with a doctor's prescription. It is a crime for anyone except a pharmacist to supply them.

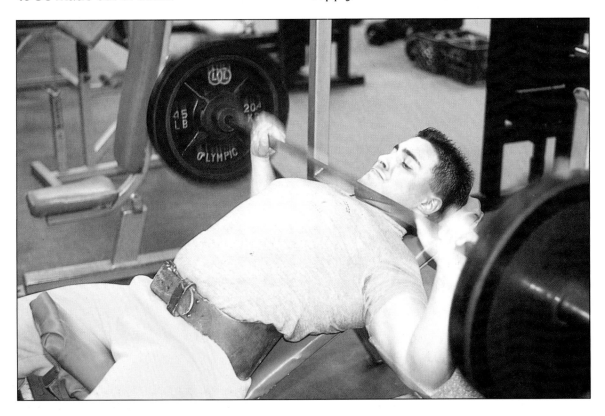

Drug dealers are attracted to gymnasiums for potential clients. Steroids enable athletes to train longer and harder and, therefore, build up strength and muscles – something many gym enthusiasts strive for.

Customs officials survey part of a drugs haul they seized when it was being smuggled from Mexico to the USA. Some of the drugs were hidden inside various art objects.

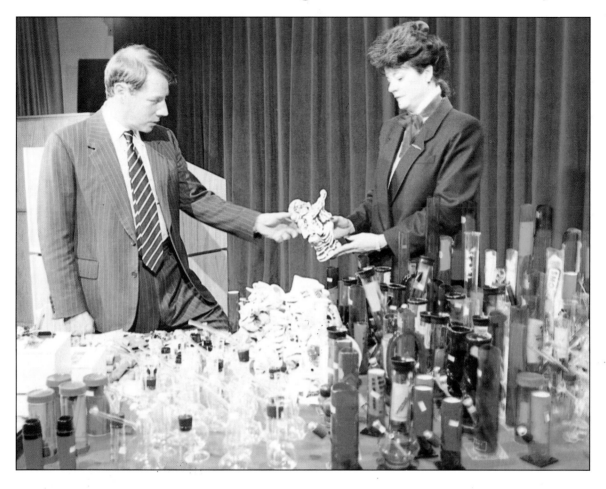

The possession of steroids for personal use is not illegal except in some US states where possession without a medical prescription has recently been made a crime. Despite the increasing criminalization, it is clear from what many athletes say, and from some investigations by journalists, that it is very easy to obtain the drugs. For example, almost every competitor in powerlifting, a non-Olympic sport similar to weightlifting but in which drug testing is not carried out, takes drugs. Books about drugs are sold at many powerlifting competitions.

A drug dealer arrested in the US in 1985 gave some idea of how the market works and how much money is made from it, *'I can't be sure but I think there may be as many as ten dealers in the US who grossed at least US $1 million dollars last year. And some do more'*. He said the dealers get it from drug manufacturing companies, drug wholesalers, or pharmacists. Pharmacists, he said, could make a lot more money supplying steroids to a few dealers than running their pharmacies. Other drugs come from Mexico, where drugs are cheap and easy

Former British track star David Jenkins (right) leaving the federal court in San Diego in 1987 after pleading guilty to directing a multi-million dollar steroid smuggling ring.

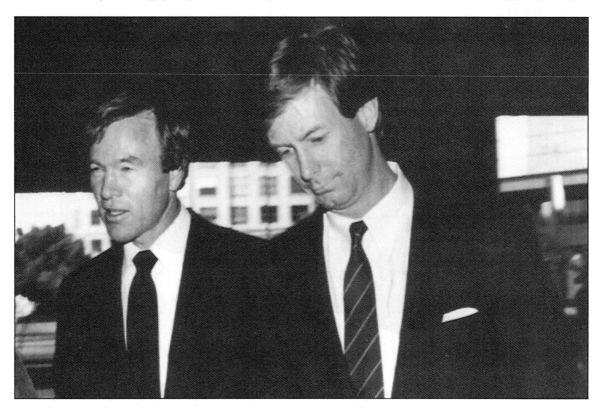

to obtain because their sale is not against the law. Most athletes buy drugs through gymnasiums. *'Every gym has at least one dealer and inside of a day you can score.'* said the same dealer. Alternatively, drugs could be obtained by mail order from advertisements in some sports magazines.

The police only began to clamp down on the dealers in the late 1980s. Before then, the authorities used to turn a blind eye or give very light sentences. For example, one dealer who was caught by customs officials in Atlanta, Georgia, with over 200,000 doses of anabolic steroids in his luggage, received only a suspended jail sentence.

The arrest of David Jenkins, a former British Olympic athlete, in Los Angeles in the late 1980s, spotlighted the way in which many former athletes are involved in the industry. Jenkins, who received a seven-year jail sentence, was convicted of having smuggled steroids from Mexico into the USA. He was part of a multi-million dollar ring involving the mass importation of drugs.

There is great concern that schoolchildren are using 'sports' drugs extensively in the USA. A survey by a professor of health education at Pennsylvania State University found that out of 3,400 boys questioned in some fifty schools in the state, 226 had used steroids. Although great care must be taken in using statistics in this way, the Pennsylvania findings suggest that as many as 250,000 adolescents could be using the drug in the USA. This figure could be higher.

In cycling races, the drugs are often provided by officials called *soigneurs, –* meaning, ironically, healer in French – who travel with the team for the whole length of the race (often as much as three weeks). The *soigneurs* look after the cyclists' medical needs. They have been referred to as *'witch-doctors, cowboys with no medical background'* by some cyclists. The soigneurs try to find out which competitors are likely to be tested at the end of each day and they give drugs to the cyclists who need them. When they are cycling seven hours a day for up to three weeks, the pressures on cyclists to take drugs are immense and the *soigneur* always has a ready supply.

In athletics, too, the teams supporting the competitors often include both doctors and coaches working closely together to find the right mix of training and 'chemical magic' to ensure victory. Ben Johnson's doctor, for example, outlined the athlete's drug programme at great length in the Canadian Government's inquiry into the affair. Having a medical team to administer the drugs makes it much easier for the athlete since the doctor can obtain supplies legally.

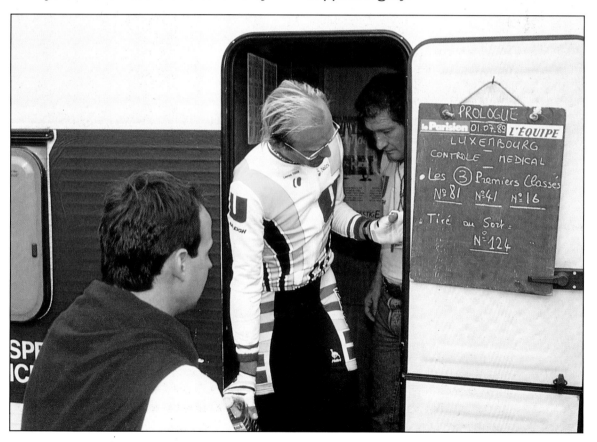

The mobile office which carries officials and medical officers around all the stages of the Tour de France.

35

CHAPTER SEVEN

TOBACCO AND ALCOHOL

THE manufacturers of the two most widely used drugs, tobacco and alcohol, provide a vast amount of money to sports events through sponsorship. Tobacco is legal in all sports, though few athletes are heavy smokers because of the damaging effects on fitness. Alcohol is banned in a few sports, such as fencing and shooting, where drunkenness could put other competitors in danger, and in winter sports, but is legal in most. However, it is unlikely to improve the performance of any competitors, though Canadian snooker player Bill Werbeniuk used to insist on drinking several litres of beer during play for what he claimed were medical reasons.

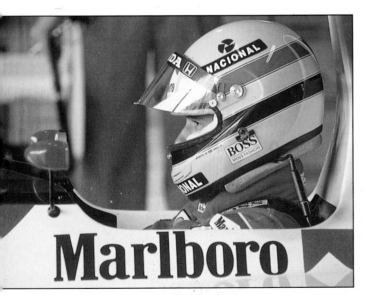

Tobacco companies get around the ban on television advertising by sponsoring sporting events which can be seen by television audiences around the world.

Both alcohol and tobacco companies sponsor a wide variety of sports. In Britain, the Tobacco Advisory Council, a lobbying group for the industry, says that £12 million per year is spent by tobacco firms on sixty different sports. A similar sum is spent on promotions to go along with sponsorship agreements, such as giving away vouchers for cheaper future purchases or advertising sponsored events. Sports sponsorship is a particularly important means of promoting cigarettes for tobacco firms – tobacco advertising on television is banned in the European Community (EC) and the USA. Tobacco firms in Britain sponsor a wide variety of sports ranging from cricket and golf to showjumping and fly fishing. In each case, the name of the event is changed to ensure that the sponsor's name is prominent, such as the Dunhill Masters (golf) and the Embassy World Snooker Championships. Advertising billboards are used at the venues to be seen by spectators and television cameras. In motor racing, cars are decorated in tobacco firms' colours and logos.

Tobacco sponsorship means that cigarette brand names often appear on the sports pages of newspapers and magazines. Effectively it gives the tobacco firms long periods of free advertising. Research by the Health Education Authority in Britain showed that in 1988 for every hour of television coverage of snooker, the sponsor's name was picked out by the camera fifteen times for an

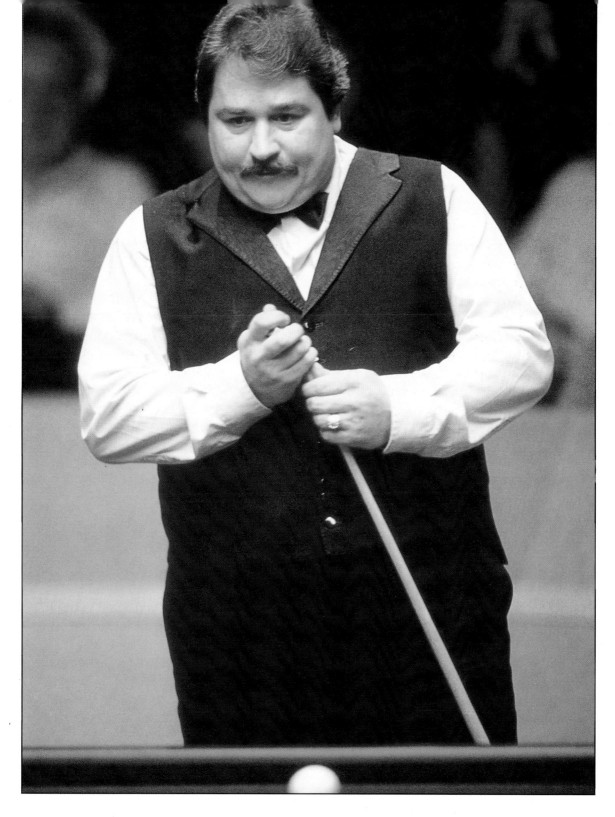

According to Canadian snooker player Bill Werbeniuk, the several litres of beer he drank during a game were for 'medical' reasons.

Many alcohol companies also manage to ensure that their brands become household names by sponsoring sports competitions.

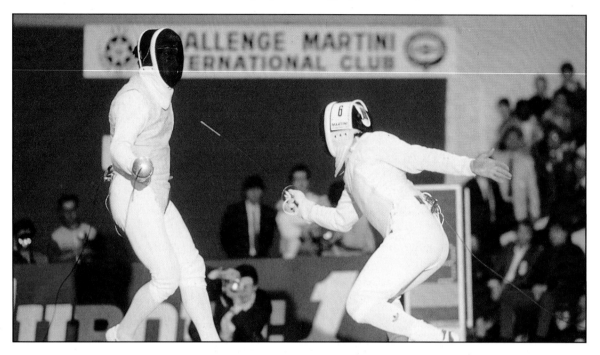

average of over seven seconds each time. This was the same as almost two minutes advertising every hour. In motor racing, where the camera follows the car, there is the name of a cigarette on the screen for as much as twenty minutes every hour. It is a very cheap form of advertising compared with the costs of buying television time. Moreover, the compulsory health warnings, such as 'tobacco kills', cannot be seen while the brand name of the cigarette clearly can. Such sponsorship is seen by its opponents as a way around the advertising ban.

This is of particular concern for the health of young people, because it is during the teenage years that people begin to smoke. Indeed, the message from sponsorship is so strong that a survey showed that 64 per cent of children aged between nine and fifteen claim to see cigarette advertising on British television. In fact, what they have seen is sport sponsored by cigarette companies because tobacco advertising is banned on television in Britain.

Tobacco firms argue that sponsorship, like advertising, is not intended to make people start smoking but is intended to advise people of the different brands on the market. However, opponents of tobacco advertising and sponsorship say that in countries where there has been a total ban, like Norway, there has been a sharp reduction in the number of people who smoke.

The alcohol industry also contributes massively to sports sponsorship. In Britain, yachting, soccer and golf benefit most from sponsorship, worth an estimated £17 million per year, plus about another £25 million in associated promotions.

There is particular concern among sporting authorities about linking alcohol closely with sport because of alcohol's role in causing hooliganism. Yet, Tottenham Hotspur and Queen's Park Rangers, two London First Division clubs, have been sponsored by alcohol companies. In 1988 the Football Association even considered allowing the FA Cup to be sponsored by an alcohol company. This is despite the fact that alcohol has been widely blamed for the Heysel disaster in Belgium in 1985. Drunken Liverpool supporters caused a riot which resulted in the death of over thirty Juventus supporters.

The link between tobacco and lung cancer and heart disease has been proved beyond doubt. Tobacco is believed to cause the death of 100,000 people per year from lung cancer and other respiratory and heart diseases in Britain, and probably three to four times that many in the USA. The harm caused by alcohol, not just to the body through disease of the liver, fatness and general ill health, but also by violent and aggressive behaviour among sports fans and in society in general, is also undeniable. Alcohol and tobacco are the two greatest causes of preventable illness. Yet, through sports' sponsorship they are associated with a healthy and beneficial life-style. It is not surprising that there is a growing number of people, both inside and outside sport, who are seeking a total ban on sponsorship by tobacco and alcohol companies. It will be interesting to see if this ever comes into effect.

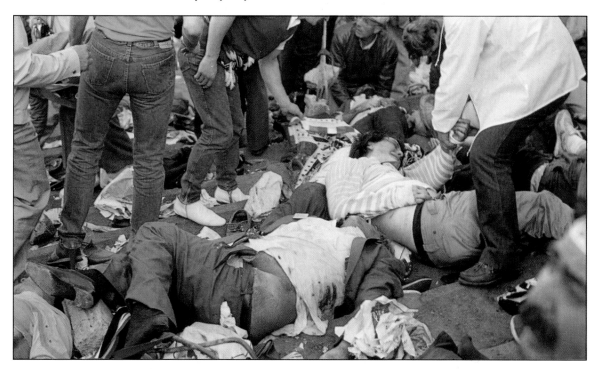

The riot that broke out during the 1985 European Cup soccer final between Liverpool and Juventus was attributed to drunken Liverpool supporters. It cost the lives of thirty people. Ironically, many soccer clubs are sponsored by alcohol companies.

CHAPTER EIGHT

EPO: THE ULTIMATE DRUG

HUMAN growth hormone or EPO (short for erythropoietin) sounds like the dream drug for athletes – amazingly effective in giving people more stamina and, so far, undetectable because it occurs naturally in the human body and therefore does not show up in tests. The only problem, which is a very serious one, is that it may have killed many sportsmen and women who have used it.

EPO is produced naturally in the human body by the kidneys and regulates the proportion of red cells in the blood.

Injecting EPO into the body increases the amount of red blood cells which is an advantage to athletes because they carry the oxygen breathed in through the lungs around the body. If you have more red cells, you can absorb more oxygen which gives you more stamina – vital for long distance runners, cyclists and skiers, for example. It has been calculated that EPO could give athletes a 10 or 12 per cent improvement, a massive help in sports where a few seconds can be the difference between first and last places.

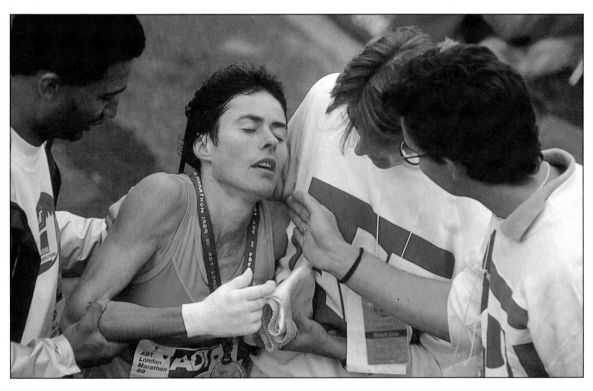

EPO occurs naturally in the human body. Some athletes from sports such as cycling, sprinting and long distance running inject EPO to increase stamina.

Stamina is very important for skiers. EPO increases the amount of red blood cells in the body and therefore more oxygen can be absorbed. The result is increased stamina.

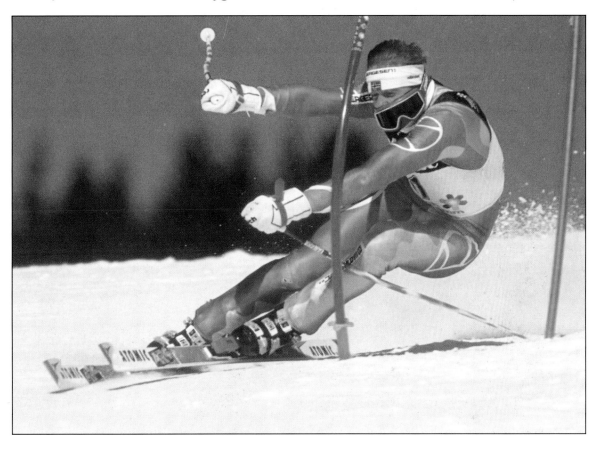

EPO has only recently become available on the market. Previously there had been no way of manufacturing the drug. Then, in the mid 1980s, a US company developed a method of synthesizing it. The drug is used medically for people suffering from a shortage of red cells, such as AIDS patients, rheumatoid arthritis sufferers and anaemics. It has been nicknamed 'go juice' because of the quick way it can increase energy.

The drug is not harmful when taken under prescription and for medical reasons but may well be harmful for athletes. Between 1987 and 1990, eighteen Dutch and Belgian cyclists died in mysterious circumstances. All were fit and healthy, without a history of heart trouble but all died suddenly from heart attacks, mostly within a couple of days of a race. Their deaths are thought to be linked to the illegal use of EPO but nothing has yet been proved conclusively.

Many of these cyclists died in the morning when the heart is least active. Doctors claim that this is because the EPO, by increasing the amount of red cells, makes the blood thicker and the heart is unable to cope with forcing thick blood through the body, causing a heart attack.

However, defenders of cycling say that the link has not been proved. They argue

Eighteen Dutch cyclists died of heart attacks between 1987 and 1990 – none, however, had any history of heart trouble. Although EPO has been put forward as the cause, there is no actual proof.

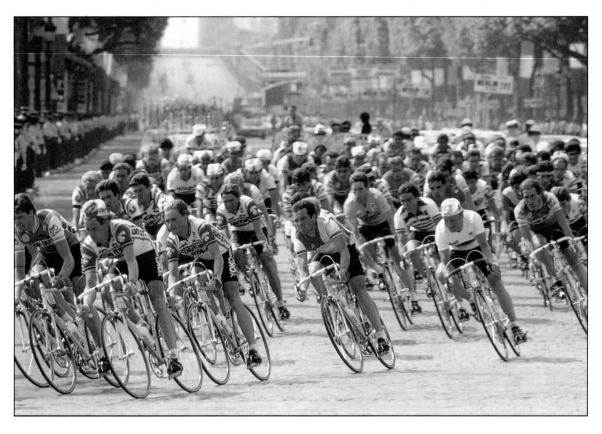

that cycling is a very hard endurance sport which often burns the body out. Many former professional cyclists, they say, die in their forties, their bodies exhausted by so many years of hard work. However, doctors point out that it was in 1987 that this mysterious set of deaths started, the same year in which EPO was first made available in both Europe and the USA. They say it is curious that the deaths have occurred in two neighbouring countries, Belgium and Holland, and suggest there may be an illegal network in which EPO is being supplied.

EPO is banned by sports authorities but as it is undetectable, this is meaningless.

The only way of detecting it would be to give all athletes regular blood tests throughout the year checking for EPO levels, but this would be very difficult to administer. Possibly the deaths of the cyclists may prove a deterrent. If a link with EPO is proved athletes may be afraid to take the drug. However, given the past history of drug use and sport, this seems unlikely. A doctor in the USA once asked over 100 runners if they would take a 'magic pill' that would guarantee them an Olympic gold medal but would kill them within the year. He found to his amazement that over half said they would take the magic pill.

CHAPTER NINE

THE DEBATE RAGES ON

THERE are two questions at the heart of the issue of sports doping. First, is using drugs cheating? Does it really matter if athletes use drugs to improve their sporting performances? Secondly, are the drugs dangerous and likely to damage those taking them?

It took a long time for sporting authorities to react to evidence that drugs were being widely used in sport. A British

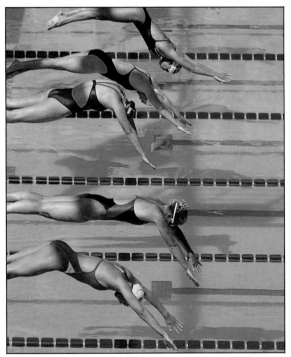

There was an obvious difference in the standard of performance of East German women swimmers before and after the merger with West Germany. It led to increased speculation about East German use of steroids.

athletics coach, Ron Pickering, says he was told to 'mind his own business' in 1964 when he tried to alert the Amateur Athletic Association to the problem. The authorities wanted to ignore the issue to avoid bad publicity and because they realized it would be a complicated and expensive issue to deal with. They were forced to recognize it by the sheer number of athletes involved and by the deaths of competitors like Tommy Simpson.

As bans began to be imposed on various drugs, doctors began to debate whether they really did improve athletes' performances and if they were harmful. It seems certain that drugs do indeed improve performances.

An interesting comparison can be made with East German swimmers after East and West Germany merged in October 1990 following the collapse of the Berlin Wall. East Germany's female swimmers had dominated the world. At the Seoul Olympics the East German women won all but one of the gold medals. Yet, just two and a half years later, at the World Championships in Perth, Australia, many of the same women could not even get into the all-German team and won only one bronze medal. In between, of course, East Germany had merged with West Germany and the very special training programmes used by the East Germans had been abandoned. Some of the former swimmers said that these programmes routinely required the use of steroids and that all the swimmers had taken them.

The likelihood that some of these drugs are harmful, is probably as strong as the link between cigarettes and bad health. Steroids, for example, are thought to cause liver and kidney problems, and have been linked with cancer. Women who take them grow beards, their voices become lower and they are unable to get pregnant. They undoubtedly make the users aggressive. As Zoe Warwicke, a British woman body builder who admits to having used steroids, put it, '...you lose friends. I was an out and out bitch when I was on steroids'. Another athlete thought he was invincible and got a friend to video his sports car as he deliberately drove into a tree to show that he was superman. Luckily he survived. However, despite all the evidence of steroids causing diseases, very few, if any, deaths have been directly linked to steroid use. In Britain, steroid use has, so far, never been put on a death certificate as the cause of death. Other drugs do seem to have been more closely related to the death of some athletes but, again, questions always remain about the exact role of drugs in causing death.

Even if drugs were shown to be entirely safe, the majority of people would still argue that they should not be used in sports. The argument is that building up your body to be the best in the world is fine if you have done it by hard training, but if it is through the use of pills, then that is cheating. One athlete put it like this, 'I believe that if I have run 5,000 m in fifteen minutes and blood-boost or injected to enable me to run it half a minute faster, then there is nothing of 'me' in that improvement'. Therefore, he says, there is nothing to be proud of. No longer can people sit back and marvel at an athlete who has just broken a world record. Instead, they must begin to question the whole ethic of sport.

British doctor Andrew Nicholson disagrees. He says, 'the amount of unfairness introduced by drug taking is no greater than that of runners using pacemakers or a few athletes having access to advanced physiological and sports medicine laboratories while the majority do not.' What is the difference, he says, between an athlete being able to afford to fly to Mexico to train at altitude and taking a little pill which may, or may not, be harmful?

Others, like Zoe Warwicke, are in the middle. She would like to see lots of measures taken to discourage the use of drugs, such as showing young people pictures of drugs users' bodies. She thinks the Sports Council is naive in wanting to impose a total ban. Large fines or even life bans would not deter people, she says. Instead, there should be widespread education on the subject.

While this debate rages on, the pressures on athletes to take drugs grows ever stronger and sports authorities try to devise more and more strict regulations. Some people are pushing for instant life bans for all those athletes found using drugs. Sport is competitive by definition and attracts people who are naturally competitive. Some athletes, as we have seen, will do anything to become the best and resort to drugs. There are no easy answers and the problem may well get worse as drugs such as EPO and other undetectable substances are discovered. There are few certainties about the use of drugs in sport, except for the fact that doping is a problem that sport will have to cope with probably for as long as there is competitive sport.

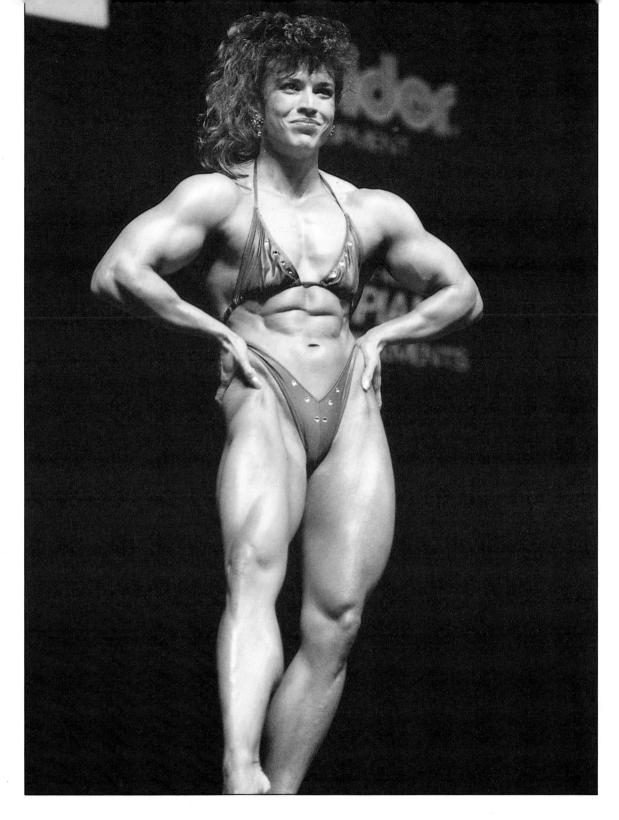

Some body builders use steroids to build up muscles. The side effects, however, can be horrific – liver and kidney problems, and possibly even cancer, for example.

GLOSSARY

Alleging Making a claim about something that is not necessarily true.

Amphetamines A group of drugs which make people more active and energetic.

Blood transfusion Injection of blood into the body, usually after loss of blood from an accident or illness.

Cannabis/Marijuana A mild illegal drug, obtained either in the form of resin or dried leaves, generally smoked, often with tobacco.

Cocaine A drug normally taken as a powder sniffed through the nose which gives a short lived effect or extra energy and can also dull pain.

Deterrent Something which deters or puts people off.

Dwarfism A medical condition which prevents growth.

Endurance Ability to withstand lengthy hardship or physical strain.

Hormones Substances, found in the body, which trigger off certain effects. Can be artificially made.

Ions Electrically charged particles.

Physiological To do with the body.

Post mortem Examination of the body after death.

Puberty Stage of growth during teenage years leading to sexual maturity.

Sponsorship Money, usually from private companies, to promote sports (or other) events.

Stimulant A drug which boosts people's energy and makes them excitable.

Unethical Contrary to normally accepted ethics of society.

FURTHER READING

Alcohol Abuse by Brian R. Ward (Franklin Watts, 1987)

Daley Thompson: The Subject is Winning by Skip Rozin (Stanley Paul, 1983)

Diet and Health by Ida Weekes (Wayland, 1991)

Drugs by Christian Wolmar (Wayland, 1990)

Drugs by Vanora Leigh (Wayland, 1986)

The Use of Drugs by Brian Ward (Macdonald, 1983)

Track Athletics by Robert Sandelson (Wayland, 1991)

The Publisher would like to establish that no person represented in this book is in any way associated with the use of drugs unless otherwise stated.

ACKNOWLEDGEMENTS

Action Plus 43, All Sport UK Ltd COVER (Yann Guichaoua), 4 (Mike Powell), 7 (Caryn Levy), 11 (Yann Guichaoua), 15 (Gray Mortimore), 17, 22, 23 (Mike Powell), 27 (top), 29, 30, 31 (Tony Duffy), 35 (Gerald Vanystadt), 36 (Pascal Rondeau), 37 (Pascal Rondeau), 39 (David Cannon), 41, 45; Mary Evans Library 5; Jeff Greenberg 32; Rex Features 16, 20 (Leo Mason), 24 (Hallalan), 26, 38 (P. Despeaux), 40 (Andrew Laenen), 42 (Rakic); Science Photo Library 9 (top, Sheila Terry), 10 (Adam Hart-Davis), 18 (Larry Mulvehill), 25 (Larry Mulvehill); Topham 6, 8, 9 (bottom), 10, 14 (Diana Wyllie), 19, 21, 27 (bottom), 28, 33, 34.

INDEX